WALKING YOUR CHILD THROUGH PUBERTY

Wendy Ologe

WALKING YOUR CHILD THROUGH PUBERTY

© 2020 Wendy Ologe

Published in Nigeria by
Smart OFFICE Ltd

For further information on permission, address:

Smart OFFICE Ltd
Suite B8, 2XL Mall, Cristiana Ajayi Okunuga Street,
3rd Avenue, Gwarimpa
Abuja, Nigeria.

Tel: +2349037163157

Email: info@smartofficeng.com

Web: www.smartofficeng.com

ISBN: 978-978-987-126-1

TABLE OF CONTENT

ACKNOWLEDGMENT

I realized that puberty is a big deal for children going through the experience since I was a child. However, when I started working with parents, it became so evident that puberty was a trying time not just for the child but for their parents as well.

It's taken me some time to get this book out, and one thing is key to note: the subject evolves daily. But it's finally out now, and I cannot be grateful enough that you have it in your hand right now.

Writing this book wouldn't have been possible if I wasn't working closely with the parents at The Intentional Parent Academy. So, I want to say thank you to them, especially the parents in our Annual Inner Circle Program who first took this course in the Academy; your push, suggestions and nudges are very much appreciated.

Thank you, Sam Gaza, for the awesome job with editing this book.

Thank you to my most cherished family: The Governor (my husband), the Twins, and our amazing foster daughter.

I am in awe of God's wonder, especially towards this work. To you the reader, without you there is no book. Thank you.

INTRODUCTION

I am sure you remember puberty, don't you? That period when your body went through a lot of changes, most of which you didn't understand or know how to respond to. Now you're the parent of a child who's experiencing these changes as well. The question is, are you going to help that child to navigate this challenging phase of his or her life effectively or will you pay no attention at all – probably as your own parents did?

In simple words, this book's goal is to show you what to expect and how you can help your child through each stage of their development and evolution into adulthood.

Sometime in 2020, we saw a spike in issues among pre-teen and teenage kids relating to their sexuality. This became obvious as the Covid-19 pandemic forced parents to become aware of the changes in their children and their own lack of knowing how to support their children through puberty. And as a response, we created a course in the online academy I lead, The Intentional Parent Academy, that helped parents to learn this all-important aspect of intentional parenting.

So far, we have had hundreds of parents take this course, and many of them reached out to ask that the lessons of the course be documented, preferably as a book, to help them easily refer to it as they walk through the puberty journey with their darling children. That request gave birth to this book. But before that, I was already developing a book I called *The Sex Conversations* which was intended to take parents through necessary and important conversations they ordinarily won't imagine having with their child when they start their puberty journey. But in honour of the requests I got, I decided to merge the developing book with the content of the course I did, thus making it even more robust and richer. So, you're in for an irrecoverable journey with this book.

Here's an email I got some time ago from a parent; perhaps you can relate with it on some level.

Good morning ma,

I stumbled on my Teen son locked up in his private restroom for long. He didn't know I was home.

When I took his phone I saw he's watching porn. He cried so much, begged, and said he has been struggling with sexual urges and masturbation.

This is a boy I raised well, has his privacy, and away from his toxic father.

He also mentioned he went to confessions according to our Catholic faith and the Priest condemned him and advised him, but he found himself there again twice, masturbating.

Please, I don't want to shame him by telling more people. He's my only child.

How do I get to help him? We cried together and prayed and he said he felt lighter.

Should I take away his phone totally?

This is one of many similar cases we receive often. But really, what happened here?

- At teenage, the puberty brain is activated and the hormones responsible for sexual urges get triggered. This is very normal.

- A teenager will experiment with a lot of things, including masturbation, especially when no one is guiding him through the teenage walks.

- This child was obviously given a phone without any form of guidance. I always advise, time and again, before you hand your child any phone, you must have a Family Media Plan. (We have a Guide that can help you build one, you can request for it).

- Puberty for the GenZ and GenAlpha child (which are the children we are raising today) is tougher! The reason is simple: they have a lot to deal with. Having one-click access to porn is one of many, for example.

Solution?

- **Kindly refer to the workbook**

Now, the most bugging question to all these is: do *you* know Show to walk your child through it all? Well, not to worry, this book will teach you all these and more. But remember, this is about caution, *not* fear! Intentional parenting is in your process; never about perfection.

Chapter 1
WHAT IS PUBERTY?

Puberty is the period during which growing boys or girls undergo the process of sexual maturation.

Puberty was awkward when you were the one going through it, remember? Now it's your child's turn; so how can you help the child through all those discomforting changes?

Puberty is a time of great change for your child – and for you as a parent, too. And it is highly important that you are very present in your child's life to support him or her through this challenging phase of their life. More so, if you do it well, chances are high that you will reap the returns for the rest of your life as you and your child will enjoy such bonding that you may not get otherwise.

To help your child, do the following to start with:

- Arm yourself with relevant and sufficient information
- Be reassuring

- Role-model body acceptance and a healthy lifestyle

- Respect your child's need for more privacy

- Take practical steps to support your child through their bodily changes

- Look after your own needs too

WHAT IS PUBERTY?

Puberty comes from the Latin word *pubertas* which means 'adult'. It's a period of life in which an individual becomes capable of sexual reproduction. There are hormones regulated by the endocrine system of the human body which lead to those physical changes. At puberty, no new hormones are produced and no new bodily system develops; the body simply utilizes what it already had to evolve the change that needs to happen within that phase.

Puberty is the period during which growing boys or girls undergo the process of sexual maturation. Puberty involves a series of physical stages or steps that lead to the achievement of fertility and the development of the so-called secondary sex characteristics, the physical features associated with adult males and females – such as the growth of pubic hair, among others.

While puberty involves a series of biological or physical transformation, the process can also have an effect on the psychosocial and emotional development of the adolescent.

Puberty education provides the cornerstone to understanding a wide range of issues concerning growth and development, self-care, relationships, body awareness, and gender differences; especially for the teenage child.

There is no other time that the human body changes more than during puberty, except during the first year of life. During this time, a major part of our self-image is formed, as well as our attitudes towards and interactions with others. So, a child will require all the support they can get from their parents or guardian in this period.

Puberty brings a lot of changes for your child – and for you as a parent, too. Your child is transitioning from child to adult, and you may feel uncertain about how best to support them through the physical, psychological and emotional changes this brings. Well, you should not fear, there's plenty you can do to help your child; you only need to learn what and how.

Puberty is simply a series of natural changes that every child goes through. Some children struggle with the changes, while others sail through puberty without concern. Only a small percentage of children experience extreme turmoil during this phase of their development, according to popular studies. But many times puberty can be exciting and special, and as your child's parent or caregiver, you're in the ideal position to help them through it.

MYTHS AND FACTS ABOUT PUBERTY

Myths about puberty can cause unnecessary anxiety in parents, so let's clear the air here. Puberty is the period of sexual maturation and achievement of fertility. Both genetic and environmental factors are involved in the timing of puberty. Body fat and/or body composition may also play a role in regulating the onset of puberty. More so, puberty is associated with the development of secondary sexual characteristics and rapid growth.

Now, let's consider some of the popular myths about puberty and counter them with facts so that you gain the right perspective and be armed to the correct information.

<u>Myth 1</u>: **Development of Pubic Hair Signals the Onset of Puberty**

<u>Fact</u>: Without breast or testicular enlargement, growth of pubic hair (pubarche) and the presence of body odor simply indicate increased adrenal secretion of weak androgens. Such changes do not signify activation of the hypothalamic-pituitary-gonadal unit (true puberty). Recent cross-sectional studies suggest that the development of pubic hair may be a normal variation in white girls as young as seven years and in black girls as young as six years. This finding alters the previous definition of premature adrenarche, which has been defined as the growth of pubic hair in girls younger than eight years and in boys younger than nine years.

<u>Myth 2</u>: **Breast Development Signals the Onset of Puberty in Girls**

<u>Fact</u>: Breast enlargement in girls younger than six years is more likely to represent benign premature thelarche than true precocious puberty.

These are the true Characteristics of Benign Premature Thelarche according to new research.

- Age younger than 6 years
- Increased breast profile
- Minimal or no growth of breast papillae (nipples) or areolae
- No growth of labia minora
- Minimal or no dulling of the vaginal mucosa, which remains shiny and reddish
- No acceleration in growth
- No pubic hair

<u>Myth 3</u>: **Pimples are a Result of Being Unclean**

<u>**Fact**</u>: Girls and boys both get pimples, and it has nothing to do with cleanliness. Instead, it's caused by hormones. It's a result of excess oil getting trapped in skin pores. Pimples usually disappear in a few days, so one shouldn't worry too much about them. Parents should make sure that pimples don't interfere with their kid's confidence. If the child feels too self-conscious about them, there are over-the-counter medication available for acne treatment that can help to clear them.

<u>Myth 4</u>: **Girls Should not be Allowed to Play During Menstruation**

<u>**Fact**</u>: Some girls may experience pain during their menstrual periods, while others may not. In either case, it should be the choice of the individual whether and how much to play. There is no reason to ask them to not touch anything while menstruating. There are many such taboos surrounding

menstruation, which forbid girls from entering the kitchen or going to a temple. These are all baseless. What matters is that you teach your girl how to keep herself clean during this period of the month and even always.

Myth 5: Menstruation is the Beginning of Puberty

Fact: Getting your period actually occurs about 18 to 24 months after puberty begins. Girls will typically get their first cycle before turning 13, but this varies in everyone; there's no rule to it.

Myth 6: Nightfall is Abnormal

Fact: Nightfall (or nocturnal emission) refers to involuntary ejaculation of semen. It's the body's way of relieving sexual arousal. When boys experience nightfall, some of them think they have a disease. Parents should reassure them that it's normal. In case it happens outdoors, for example, in a movie theatre during a kissing scene, boys can just head to the restroom and clean themselves up.

<u>Myth 7</u>: **Menstrual Blood is Impure**

<u>Fact</u>: Menstruation is an absolutely natural process. Scientifically speaking, menstrual discharge does not contain any toxic components. About half of menstrual fluid is blood. Other components include calcium, iron, sodium, cervical mucus, etc. It is no more dangerous than regular blood.

<u>Myth 8</u>: **Something is Wrong If Kids Don't Grow Taller Soon After Puberty Hits**

<u>Fact</u>: The growth period for everyone varies. Parents should not worry if their children are not as tall as their classmates or other kids in the neighborhood, or if they don't have muscles. Boys normally see an increase in height between the ages of 12 to 16 or 18, while for girls it's normally between 9 to 15.

Other Facts (culled from the American Family Physician portal)

Girls go through puberty at a younger age if their father isn't present in their lives, and some risk has been found to be associated with early puberty

- Central Precocious Puberty (CPP) is puberty that occurs earlier than normal due to release of hormones from the hypothalamus of the brain

- Girls are more likely than boys to have precocious puberty (early puberty)

- Breast development is usually the first sign of puberty in girls

- Puberty may also be accompanied by emotional and mood changes

- Some medical conditions may worsen or first become apparent at puberty

- Precocious puberty is defined as the onset of true puberty before 8 years of age in girls or 9 years of age in boys

- Isolated breast development that doesn't progress to the rest of puberty is called premature thelarche and is a different, benign condition

- Precocious puberty is 10 times more common in girls than in boys. Sexual development may begin at any age

- Pregnancy has been reported as early as 5½ years old

- The Lawson Wilkins Pediatric Endocrine Society recommends evaluating for an underlying medical condition in Caucasian-American girls who have development of breast and/or pubic hair before age seven and in African-American girls before age six. These medical conditions include tumors, cysts, thyroid problems, McCune-Albright syndrome, or external sources of estrogen. Doing studies to look into these possible causes is especially important in girls younger than 6, and in all boys

- The earlier before age 12 a girl starts her period, the higher her lifetime risk for breast cancer (probably from the prolonged estrogen exposure). The highest average risk for breast cancer is in non-Hispanic white women, where it is 1 in 8, or 12.5%. In all girls who start their periods before the age of 12, taken together, the risk is 16.25%.

- As a girl reaches maturity, she needs to be made aware of controllable risk factors for breast cancer, such as use of estrogen-containing birth control pills (10 years of use would raise her risk to about 22%), first pregnancy after age 30 (if she did this also, it would raise the risk to about 35%), high-fat diet, alcohol use, fertility drugs, pesticides, and radiation exposure. Each of these factors multiplies her accumulated risk.

When Does Puberty Start?

Doctors do not completely understand the timing of the onset of puberty; a number of factors likely determine its onset. One theory proposes that reaching a critical weight or body composition may play a role in the onset of puberty. The increase in childhood obesity may be related to the overall earlier onset of puberty in the general population in recent years, some experts suggest.

Leptin, a hormone produced by fat cells (adipocytes) in the body, has been suggested as one possible mediator of the timing of puberty. In research studies, animals deficient in leptin did not undergo puberty, but puberty began when leptin was administered to the animals. Further, girls with higher concentrations of the leptin hormone are known to have an increased percentage of body fat and an earlier onset of puberty than girls with lower levels of leptin. The concentration of leptin in the blood is known to increase just before puberty in both boys and girls.

Leptin, however, is likely only one of multiple influences on the hypothalamus, an area of the brain that releases a hormone known as gonadotropin-releasing hormone (GnRH), which in turn signals the pituitary gland to release luteinizing hormone (LH) and follicle-stimulating hormone (FSH). LH and FSH secretion by the pituitary is responsible for sexual development through regulation of the production of estrogen and testosterone.

Genetic factors are likely involved in the timing of puberty, and the timing of puberty tends to "run in families." Additionally, a gene has been identified that appears to be critical for the normal development of puberty. The gene, known as GPR54, encodes a protein that appears to have an effect on the secretion of GnRH by the hypothalamus. Individuals who do not have a functioning copy of this gene are not able to enter puberty normally.

Overall, no two people are exactly alike, but one thing everyone has in common is that we all go through puberty, irrespective of what time it starts for each person. Usually, puberty starts between ages 8 and 13 in girls and ages 9 and 15 in boys.

One day your daughter is asking about when her period starts or your son comes home from school or the playground smelling in an offensive manner ... What's going on? Welcome to puberty, the time when children sprout up, fill out, and maybe even mouth off.

Effects of Puberty Timing

With a few exceptions, pubertal timing – that is, early or late maturation – appeared associated with other problems than tanner stage in itself. Early maturing adolescents felt lonelier, as evidenced by feelings of being unloved and inferior, thoughts about killing self, or running away from home.

This is conceivable considering that deviation from normative timing implies a lack of same-aged friends to discuss one's changing body with (A preference for older kids fits into that picture). Late maturers tend to have fewer problems than early maturers, or, at least they experience fewer significant effects. Perhaps this is because late maturing adolescents can anticipate and adapt to the changes while observing earlier maturing peers. However, it may also be due to the lower power to detect differences in this group. Most likely, symptoms that are associated with the timing of puberty are more transient than symptoms associated with maturation itself or with age. Early maturers also, reportedly, exhibit more uncontrolled behaviors such as temper tantrums and destroying things. This could be the result of the unfortunate combination of puberty-related hormonal perturbations with a relatively immature brain.

How Long Does Puberty Take?

The process has no predetermined onset or length. Timing varies widely and can be influenced by a wide range of environmental factors and cues that are not entirely known. "Normal" puberty onset can range from ages 8 – 13 and take, on average, 1.5 – 6 years to complete.

Most experts agree that the decline in the age of puberty is attributable to decreased rates of disease, increased nutrition, and humans' ability to adapt sexual maturation to environmental cues such as health, food, shelter. This is why it is difficult to speak of a "normal" age and time for puberty. We are adaptive creatures and "normal" depends upon our personal and communal conditions. This also means that "normal" puberty development is not necessarily "good" or "healthy;" it's simply an average marker of response to external circumstances that impact internal functions.

Signs of Puberty

Sure, most of us know the telltale signs of puberty like hair growth in new places, menstruation, body odor, lower voice in boys, breast growth in girls, etc.

Usually, after a girl's 8th birthday or after a boy turns 9 or 10, puberty begins when an area of the brain called the hypothalamus starts to release gonadotropin-releasing hormone (GnRH). When GnRH travels to the pituitary gland (a small gland under the brain that produces hormones that control other glands throughout the body), it releases two more puberty hormones: luteinizing hormone (LH) and follicle-stimulating hormone (FSH).

What happens next depends on gender:

<u>Boys</u>

Hormones travel through the bloodstream to the testes (testicles) and give the signal to begin production of sperm and the hormone testosterone. At about the same time, the adrenal glands of both boys and girls begin to produce a group of hormones called adrenal androgens. These hormones stimulate the growth of pubic and underarm hair in both sexes.

The physical changes of puberty for a boy usually start with enlargement of the testicles and sprouting of pubic hair, followed by a growth spurt between ages 10 and 16 – on average 1 to 2 years later than when girls start. His arms, legs, hands and feet also grow faster than the rest of his body. His body shape will begin to change as his shoulders broaden and he gains weight and muscles.

A boy may become concerned if he notices tenderness or swelling under his nipples. This temporary development of breast tissue is called gynecomastia and it happens to about 50% of boys during puberty. But it usually disappears within 6 months or so.

And that first crack in the voice is a sign that his voice is changing and will become deeper. Dark, coarse, curly hair will also sprout just above his penis and on his scrotum, and later under his arms and in the beard area. His penis and testes will get larger, and erections, which a boy begins experiencing as an infant, will become more frequent. Ejaculation – the release of sperm-containing semen – will also occur.

Many boys become concerned about their penis size. A boy may need reassurance, particularly if he tends to be a later developer and he compares himself with boys who are further along in puberty. If a boy is circumcised, he may also have questions about the skin that covers the tip of an uncircumcised penis.

Girls

Puberty generally starts earlier for girls, sometime between 8 and 13 years of age. For most girls, the first evidence of puberty is breast development, but it can be the growth of pubic hair. As her breasts start to grow, a girl will initially have small, firm, tender lumps (called buds) under one or both nipples. The breast tissue will get larger and become less firm in texture over the next year or two. Dark, coarse, curly hair will appear on her labia (the folds of skin surrounding the vagina), and later, similar hair will begin growing under her arms.

The first signs of puberty are followed 1 or 2 years later by a noticeable growth spurt. Her body will begin to build up fat, particularly in the breasts and around her hips and thighs, as she takes on the contours of a woman. Her arms, legs, hands and feet will also get bigger.

The culminating event will be the arrival of menarche, her first period (menstruation). Depending on the age at which they begin their pubertal development, girls may get their first period between the ages of 9 and 16.

Why Does Puberty Happen?

When a child's body is ready to begin puberty, pituitary gland (a pea-shaped gland located at the bottom of the brain) releases special hormones. Depending on whether they're a boy or a girl, these hormones go to work on different parts of the body.

During puberty, the body becomes able to reproduce, or have children. The reproductive parts mature and the body grows bigger and stronger. The child's brain also matures and helps them to make new social connections.

Chapter 2
STAGES OF PUBERTY?

Professor James M. Tanner, a child development expert, was the first to identify the visible stages of puberty. These are known as tanner stage, or sexual maturity ratings today. They serve as a general guide to physical development.

According to Rena Goldman in her article on healthline.com (Healthline Media a Red Ventures Company) as Medically reviewed by Karen Gill, M.D. These are what happens at the Tanner stages.

TANNER STAGE 1

This is also known as pre-pubertal stage; At this stage there are no physical signs as it's the period that ushers in physical changes. Toward the end of stage 1, the brain is just starting to send signals to the body to prepare for changes.

- The hypothalamus begins to release gonadotropin-releasing hormone (GnRH), which then travels to the pituitary gland, the small area under the brain that produces hormones that control other glands in the body.

- The pituitary gland produces and releases two other hormones: luteinizing hormone (LH) and follicle-stimulating hormone (FSH).

- These early signals typically start after a girl's 8th birthday and after a boy's 9th or 10th birthday. There aren't any noticeable physical changes for boys or girls at this stage.

How Children React Emotionally to this Stage

- A child's self-awareness and self-concept undergo profound development during the puberty period, and it starts now – at this stage.

- At this stage children begin to see the perceived opinions of peers as important. This will shape their self-concept and modulate their social behavior going forward.

- At this stage, the ability to feel mixed emotions starts. Children below 8 years rarely understand this concept; only between the ages of 10 and 11 are children able to describe situations in which two opposite valence emotions would be felt simultaneously.

- This typically means your child might feel different emotions about their body; and if they have never been taught how to name their emotions, they might not be able to accurately describe how they feel.

TANNER STAGE 2

This marks the beginning of physical development. Hormones begin to send signals throughout the body.

<u>In Girls</u>

- Puberty usually starts between ages 8 and 11. The first signs of breasts, called 'buds,' start to form under the nipple. They may be itchy or tender, which is normal.

- It's common for breasts to be different sizes and grow at different rates. So, it's normal if one bud appears larger than the other. The darker area around the nipple (areola) will also expand.

- In addition, the uterus begins to get larger, and small amounts of pubic hair start growing on the lips of the vagina.

- On average, African girls start puberty a year before Caucasian girls, and are ahead when it comes to breast development and having their first periods. Also, girls with higher body mass index experience an earlier onset of puberty.

In Boys

In boys, puberty usually starts around age 11. The testicles and skin around the testicles (scrotum) begin to get bigger. Also, early stages of pubic hair form on the base of the penis.

<u>**How Children React Emotionally to this Stage**</u>

- Children in early to mid-puberty are more self-conscious than both pre-pubescent children and post-pubescent adolescents.

- It has been suggested that the physical changes of puberty contribute to developmentally enhanced self-consciousness, through a mechanism of heightened vulnerability to environmental circumstances that threaten the child's self-image (Simmons et al., 1973).

  - Thus, mid-puberty may be a time of particular sensitivity to social or self-conscious emotions such as embarrassment and shame.

TANNER STAGE 3

Physical changes are becoming more obvious.

Physical changes in girls usually start after age 12. They include:

- Breast 'buds' continue to grow and expand

- Pubic hair gets thicker and curlier

- Hair starts forming under the armpits

- The first signs of acne may appear on the face and back

- The highest growth rate for height begins (around 3.2 inches per year)

- Hips and thighs start to build up fat

Physical changes in boys usually start around age 13 and include:

- Penis gets longer as testicles continue to grow bigger

- Some breast tissue may start to form under the nipples (this happens to some teenage boys during development and usually goes away within a couple of years)
- Boys begin to have wet dreams (ejaculation at night)
- As the voice begins to change, it may 'crack,' going from high to lower pitches
- Muscles get larger
- Height growth increases to 2 to 3.2 inches per year

TANNER STAGE 4

Puberty is in full swing during stage 4. Both boys and girls are experiencing many changes in their bodies, both physically and internally.

In girls, stage 4 usually starts around age 13 and the changes include:

- Breasts take on a fuller shape, passing the bud stage
- Many girls get their first period, typically between the ages of 12 and 14, but it can happen earlier

- Height growth will slow down to about 2 to 3 inches per year
- Pubic hair gets thicker

In boys, stage 4 usually starts around age 14. Changes include:

- Testicles, penis, and scrotum continue to get bigger, and the scrotum will get darker in color
- Armpit hair starts to grow
- Deeper voice becomes permanent
- Acne may start to appear

TANNER STAGE 5

This final phase marks the end of your child's physical maturation.

In girls, stage 5 usually happens around age 15. The changes they undergo include:

- Breasts reach approximate adult size and shape, although breasts can continue to change through to age 18
- Periods become regular after six months to two years
- Girls reach adult height one to two years after their first period
- Pubic hair fills out to reach the inner thighs
- Reproductive organs and genitals are fully developed
- Hips, thighs, and buttocks fill out in shape

In boys, stage 5 usually starts around age 15, introducing the following changes:

- Penis, testicles, and scrotum will have reached adult size
- Pubic hair has filled in and spread to the inner thighs
- Facial hair will start growing out and some boys will need to begin shaving
- Growth in height will slow down, but muscles may still be growing
- By age 18 most boys have reached full growth

ATTITUDES AND CHARACTERS THAT MAY INCREASE WITH TANNER STAGES

<u>Internalizing problems</u>

- Secretive, keep things to themselves

- Underactive

- Lack of energy

- Overtired without obvious reason

- Feel dizzy or light-headed often

- Too shy or timid

- Unhappy, sad, or depressed

- Self-conscious, easily embarrassed, worry a lot

<u>Externalizing problems</u>

- Stubborn

- Irritable

- Mean to others

- Disobedient at home

- Disobedient at school

- Unusually loud

- Thinks about sex too much

- Breaks rules and boundaries

- Prefers being with older kids

- Steals outside the home

- Truancy

- Swears, uses obscene language

- Drinks alcohol without permission

- Smokes/chews tobacco or takes snuffs

- Uses drugs

- Screams a lot

- Mood changes/swings

Attitudes that may Decrease with Tanner Stages

- Fear of certain animals or situations

- Fear of going to school

- Being too fearful or anxious

- Stomach aches or cramps

- Teasing behaviour

- Crying a lot

- Feeling (s)he has to be perfect

- Feeling worthless or inferior

- Nervous, high-strung, tense

  Feeling too guilty

- Nausea, feeling sick often

- Hangs around with others who get in trouble

What to Expect from Your Child During Puberty – Socially and Emotionally

- Mood changes and energy level variations are normal parts of puberty, as are swings between feeling independent and wanting parental support.

- Your child will want to establish their own identity, which may include new friendships and experiences.

If this happens, they will encounter challenges with how to manage current friendships. They may also start to explore their sexuality and may go on dates and start developing romantic relationships.

- Puberty and adolescence is a time for children to become more independent They may also be looking for more responsibility, such as taking on a leadership position at school or finding a part-time job.

- Your child may also be sensitive about how they look and their new body changes. Privacy and personal space may become very important to them. They may alternate between feeling self-conscious about themselves one day to feeling 'bulletproof' the next.

- These social and emotional changes show your child is forming their own identity and learning how to be an independent adult. They are developing their decision-making skills and learning to recognize and understand the consequences of their actions.

- Change can feel strange. Just as those hormones change the way your child's body looks on the outside, they also create changes on the inside. During puberty, your child might feel confused or have strong emotions that they've never had before. They might feel overly sensitive or become upset easily. Some children lose their tempers more often and get angry with their friends or families. They may also feel anxious about how their changing body looks.

Sometimes it can be hard to deal with all these new emotions. It's important to know that as their body is adjusting to the new hormones, so is their mind. Try to remember to assure your child that people usually aren't trying to hurt their feelings or upset them on purpose – it's just their new "puberty brain" trying to adjust.

Again, your child might have sexual feelings that they've never felt before. And they will probably have lots of questions about these new, confusing feelings about sex. So, while it's likely that you would feel embarrassed or uneasy about talking sex with your child, it's important to get their questions answered, but you need to be sure you have all the right information first. That's why, to help you equip adequately ahead, I have added some common questions your child might ask at this stage in their life; and if they are not asking, I have also provided conversation starters to help you initiate the conversation.

What to Remember and Expect During Puberty

I.   The changes of puberty are physical, sexual, social and emotional. Puberty starts when changes in your child's brain cause sex hormones to be released in the ovaries (usually around age 10 or 11, but can range from 8 to 13 years), or testes (usually around ages 11 to 13, but can range from 9 to 14 years).

II.   You can't predict how long your child will go through puberty. It may be anywhere from 18 months up to 5 years.

III.   Genetic, nutritional and social factors determine

when puberty starts and for how long it runs.

IV.   During puberty, most children will experience:

- Oily skin (acne is possible)

- Oily hair, possibly requiring frequent washing

- Increased perspiration and body odour (frequent

showering and deodorant will help to manage this)

- A growth spurt (of around 11 cm a year in girls and up

to 13 cm a year in boys). Teens continue to grow about

1-2 cm a year after this main growth spurt. Some

body parts (such as head and hands) may grow faster

than limbs and torso, but the body eventually evens

out.

Remember, at each of these stages your child will need you to be present with knowledge and lots of encouragement.

Chapter 3
UNDERSTANDING YOUR CHILD

THE PUBERTY BRAIN

Researchers have discovered that puberty not only changes the body, it also changes the brain. This is because puberty involves changes in hormones that also attach to brain cells and change how the brain learns and grows. These changes are useful because they help shape the brain for new forms of learning. They might also lead to some "bumps in the road," like you might take some risks that do not quite work out.

In this chapter we will explain what puberty does to the brain and why these brain changes are important to prepare your child for adulthood.[1] But then, what exactly happens in the body to cause these changes?

The brain signals the body to start puberty by passing along messages in the form of hormones, which are small messengers that travel in the bloodstream to various parts of the body. Testosterone and estradiol are two hormones that are important for puberty.

Hormones are small molecules produced by the human body and travel in the bloodstream to various parts of the body, including the brain. Hormones are important for passing messages over long distances in the body, so that different organs can communicate with each other. When a hormone reaches its destination, it attaches to what is called a receptor – a structure in or on a cell that a hormone or other messenger can attach to. This triggers a response in the cell that can influence the cell's behavior and even its survival.

Hormones Can Change How Brain Cells Behave

Hormones like testosterone and estradiol can attach to your brain cells. A brain cell looks different from cells in other parts of the body: it has a cell body, but also has parts that look like wires sticking out. A brain cell often has many short "wires," called dendrites, which are the parts that receive signals from other cells. They also have one longer "wire" called an axon, which sends signals to other cells.

There are two main ways that hormones can influence your brain cells.

First, hormones can influence how the brain is organized, and these are changes that take some time to occur. Changes in brain organization can include changes in the number of cells or changes in the size and shape of dendrites or axons. Testosterone, for example, influences the development of new cells in a brain region called the medial amygdala which is a small region near the bottom of the brain that is important for processing emotions, like fear.

Secondly, a hormone can influence the way that brain cells become activated in response to a situation or environment. Hormones might help or prevent a cell from exchanging signals with other cells. This can also lead to long-term changes in brain cells. For example, the levels of testosterone in mice (and humans) increase during a competition or fight.

How Does This Affect Learning?

Puberty may make it harder to learn some things, but easier to learn others.

Children can learn certain things better than teenagers or adults can. For example, young children are particularly good at learning new languages. It becomes much harder to learn a second language after a person is 9–11 years old. This is probably because of changes in the way the brain processes speech and other language information.

One study looked at the role of puberty in these changes. The researchers let children listen to speech from a fake "alien" language and studied how the brain tried to make sense of this. The activity in several brain regions important for language changed as children got older. Activity in some of these language-related brain regions was also lower for children who were further along in puberty. This suggests that puberty plays a role in the brain's changing responses to language.

However, puberty might open a window for other types of learning. It might bring opportunities for learning about oneself and learning social and emotional skills that prepare teenagers for adulthood. The brain might change during the teenage years in ways that support such learning.

As an example, one important part of learning new skills is responding to feedback; that is, how your brain uses information telling you whether or not you have gotten the right answer. One study of over 200 children, teenagers, and adults looked at how the brain responds when learning from feedback. How well people learned from feedback was related to activation in different parts of the striatum – an area in the middle of the brain that processes rewards and feedback. It is called the striatum because the alternating types of tissues there make it look striped, and it is a key brain region for learning. Some parts of the striatum were more active in teenagers than in children or adults, suggesting that people might learn from feedback differently during their teenage years.

Another important part of learning new skills requires exploration and risks, like sharing information about yourself, trying out a new hobby that you might not be good at, or trying to talk to someone you have a crush on. Deciding to take a risk might be more likely when you think you have something to gain – like a reward.

Scientists have seen that part of the striatum also activates when a person receives rewards, including food and money. One study of people between ages 8-27 focused on this brain region. The researchers found that people who were further along in puberty and people who had more testosterone in their bodies showed more activation in this part of the striatum when winning a reward. This suggests that hormones may be important for making your brain more sensitive to reward during puberty.[2]

These studies show that the way the brain responds to feedback and rewards changes around puberty. This may encourage teenagers to learn more about themselves and others, supporting self-discovery and personal growth. However, these brain changes might also be related to the reality that certain mental health problems and drug addictions tend to develop during the teenage years. For example, if teenagers are more sensitive to rewards, they might also be more sensitive to the perceived rewarding feeling that comes with taking alcohol or a drug. Also, children who go through puberty earlier or faster than their peers can have more mental health struggles, which researchers think could be partly due to hormones having a different impact on their brains.

These changes might be important for opening up new opportunities for learning that prepare teenagers for adulthood, although the same brain changes might also close windows for other types of learning that happen earlier in childhood. Schools might be able to take advantage of these brain changes in their students, for instance by creating opportunities for positive forms of exploration and risk taking. Learning is more than math and reading; making decisions that help us to better understand ourselves and others is another important kind of learning that the brain might be especially sensitive to during puberty.

Behavior, Problem Solving, and Decision Making

Many parents do not understand why their teenagers occasionally behave in an impulsive, irrational, or dangerous way. At times, it seems like teens don't think things through or fully consider the consequences of their actions. Adolescents differ from adults in the way they behave, solve problems, and make decisions. There is a biological explanation for this difference. Studies have shown that brains continue to mature and develop throughout childhood and adolescence and well into early adulthood.

Which Part of Their Brain Do Teenagers Use Most of the Time?

Experiments have been done to show that teens often 'think with their feelings'. Scans of the brain can be done to show different parts lighting up when they are being used. When adults and teens look at faces showing different emotions, the parts of their brains that light up are different. Adults use their prefrontal cortex to look at faces and try to decide what emotion is happening. Teenagers use their amygdala rather than their prefrontal cortex most of the time. In other words, they are using their emotions to try and understand expressed emotions.

To understand how this feels, imagine you have lost your car keys and you are already late for work. Think about how many times you look for the keys in the same place – 5, 10, even 20 times. You panic – you no longer think with your cortex; you are thinking with your emotions. Remember how it feels if someone tells you to calm down and think sensibly about when you last had them. That is how your teenager feels when they are running on their emotions, because their brain hasn't developed that linkage to reasoning detached from emotion yet.

Oftentimes teens can misinterpret emotions. They see anger when in reality you are feeling anxious. This can often lead to many moments of miscommunication. So, when you are talking to teenagers, be careful to check what emotion they are seeing in you and make sure you always acknowledge their emotions first, and then help them to be able to think about what they are feeling.

Based on the stage of their brain development, adolescents are more likely to:

- Act on impulse
- Misread or misinterpret social cues and emotions
- Get into accidents of all kinds
- Get involved in fights
- Engage in dangerous or risky behavior

Adolescents are less likely to:

- Think before they act
- Pause to consider the consequences of their actions
- Change their dangerous or inappropriate behaviors

These brain differences don't mean that young people can't make good decisions or tell the difference between right and wrong. It also doesn't mean that they shouldn't be held responsible for their actions. However, an awareness of these differences can help parents, teachers, to understand, anticipate, and manage the behavior of adolescents.

What Can Help Brain Development During Puberty?

The brain is thought to develop and connect functionally in stages. The emotional areas of the brain (the limbic system) are present at birth, but regulation of emotions moves from being more of a shared responsibility (with parents) in childhood, to an individual responsibility in adolescence. This process requires new connections to be formed between the cortical or higher level thinking and the emotional areas of the brain. It also leads to adult level decision making, planning and thinking. The following are ways to help your teenage child's brain to develop effectively.

- **Talk to Your Child**: Adults (parents) who talk to children as they are growing up really help.

- **A Safe Environment**: A safe environment where they have consistent, loving support is vital for the brain to develop well. Young people need adults to believe in them and encourage them.

- **The Discipline That Works**: Teenagers respond better to guidance and rewards than to punishment. They need clear, consistent boundaries; and very importantly, their growing capacity and ability to do things independently need to be respected. In my book. *The Discipline that Works*, I share strategies that can help you learn effective discipline.

- **Independence**: As their brain grows and gets connected functionally, they need to learn that they don't have to be dependent on their parents but can become interdependent with other adults as they mature. They need opportunities to grow many different skills and to contribute those skills in a way that is valued. The brain develops in a way that produces lots of connections that are then removed if they are not used. So take care to encourage lots of connections to be used.

What Harms the Development of the Puberty Brain?

- **Abuse**: It is now well established that if children experience any sort of abuse (verbal, emotional, physical, sexual or neglect), especially in the early years of life, it can affect how the brain is wired and functions. Sometimes this is hard to change, so it is very important to protect children throughout their development. This is especially important at times of peak brain development during pregnancy and the first 5 years of life and during the second phase of brain development around puberty.

- **Alcohol and Drugs**: Alcohol and drugs (such as methamphetamine) can be poisonous to the developing brain, particularly during pregnancy and adolescence. Even one drink can cause a lot of damage at certain times of brain development. During adolescence, existing connections between brain cells are strengthened and set for life. Alcohol and drug use during this stage can affect memory and organization. For optimal brain development, it is best to avoid alcohol until adulthood.

How Relationships Affect the Puberty Brain

Fact 1 – Families matter: Adolescents who have a positive relationship with their parents are less likely to start sexual intercourse early.

Fact 2 – Friends matter: Adolescents who believe that their friends are sexually active are more likely to start sexual intercourse early.

Researchers' findings show that teenage boys really are motivated by love and a desire for meaningful relationships. Boys are constantly in need of who to talk to somebody, but they can't talk to their boy-friends because it's all teasing and a lot of competitiveness.

Fact 3 - Beliefs matter: Adolescents who have spiritual beliefs are less likely to start sexual intercourse early.

What to Note:

Risk behaviours are linked. Adolescents who engage in risk behaviours such as using alcohol and drugs are more likely to start sexual intercourse early.

Chapter 4
PORN LITERACY

In this chapter you will learn why it is highly important for you to discuss the vital subject of pornography with your child, especially because of the times we live, and how to go about it.

One of the defining characteristics of puberty is an increase in gonadal steroid hormone secretion, which not only fuels sexual feelings and motivation but may also change the nature of sensory organs, sexual feelings and motivation, experiences and autonomic (re)activity, especially when the body is still adjusting to the changes and hormone cycles may be irregular.

The increase in reported sexual thoughts and behaviors and in irritability found in researches seems to be a logical consequence of these hormonal developments. Likewise, the increase in tiredness could result from the adjustment to changing hormone concentrations. And the fact that these symptoms were not just associated with Tanner stage, but also with age suggests that socio-cultural factors (e.g., peer behaviors) play a role as well.

Today, we must educate children about both sex and porn. I am now advocating that pornography should be taught as part of sex education in schools. Porn literacy teaches children to define pornographic terms that are problematic, discuss sexting, sexual/gender/dating violence, and to question the industry as a whole. We cannot continue raising a generation of children who either feel wildly awkward discussing the issue or believe that it is realistic and enter relationships having expectations that will never be met. Pornography is a business that will probably never cease to exist, but the way we teach porn literacy has to.

I read this Article sometime ago about Porn targeting children through video games by Steve Warren.

The World's Largest Porn Company is Targeting Your Children Through Video Games by Steve Warren

Porn is tightening its grip on many children through two major areas – online gaming and virtual reality.

As recently as five years ago, the number of video games containing pornographic sexual violence was minimal, according to Ben Miller, digital strategies coordinator for the National Center on Sexual Exploitation (NCOSE). But now, the center reports the numbers of these games are skyrocketing.

Last year, one popular video game website hosted 780 games with nudity. This year, the same website hosts more than 1,600 of these games.

Now, a company that owns a large number of top porn studios and websites has started a distribution platform for online pornographic games.

"Porn games don't simply contain sex and nudity. Rather, they are much more graphic," Miller said in a press release. "Some of these games promote sexual harassment and assault. Despite being cartoons, the graphic content in these games is far from harmless. Animated porn fuels sexual addiction and shapes sexual palettes just as regular porn does."

The provider's website traffic has exploded from 50 million to 115 million visits between April and August 2018, ranking it in the top 500 websites in the world.

Parents need to be aware of the impact the increase in pornographic online gaming may have on their children.

"Parents need to understand how intricately linked the gaming industry and pornography industry are,". "More and more games have pornography embedded in them. If children play online, that is a pornographer's heyday for marketing, grooming, and hooking young consumers."

Virtual Reality (VR) is also a booming business.

Another major adult gaming portal announced last May that it is expanding into virtual reality with two new VR products. Through the use of a headset such as the Oculus Rift (owned by Facebook), a viewer can enter a manufactured environment and tune out the reality of their actual situation.

Fortune Magazine stated, "By 2025, adult virtual reality content is forecast to be a $1 billion business, the third biggest sector behind video games and NFL-related content, according to Piper Jaffray analyst Travis Jakel."

Todd Glider, CEO of VR adult entertainment company BaDoink, said: "VR will become the standard in the industry for today's younger male consumers."

"I see it through a generational lens. VR porn will not have a pronounced effect on the demographic born before 1980," he continued. "However, for the generations born after, the ones that reach adulthood in a world where 24/7 access to adult content is just a mouse click away, that's the audience for VR porn, and it will be huge."

Here are some steps you can take to protect your children:

- Keep the gaming device or computer in a high-traffic area, not in the child's room, even if you already have an internet filter service.

- Remove the headphones and make them use the computer's speakers so you can hear any online chatting.

- Set up all of your children's game accounts and console controls. You decide who has access to their gaming profile and who your child can talk to.

- Learn how to use the parental controls that are built into the console. Read reviews and understand the industry rating system.

- Make sure the game is age-appropriate. Talk to your children. Teach them basic internet safety roles and to notify you if they encounter anything unusual or unsettling while they are playing.

- a non-shaming relationship with your child so that if they do come across adult content, they can approach you and talk about it.

Is Porn Addictive?

When we watch porn, a chemical called dopamine is released in our brain, which makes us feel good. We naturally want to keep going back to porn to get this feeling, and we soon start to crave more of it. Once we've started, it can be difficult to stop. Some young people who watch a lot of porn describe an inability to stop, even when their porn use is impacting their school work, friendships, social life, or partner. In a recent NZ study of young people, according to www.healthnavigator.org.nz, 42% admitted 'they would like to watch less porn but find it hard not to'. Some young people also find their preference for the type of porn changes with the more they watch – and they need increasingly violent and extreme porn in order to get aroused. There are a number of neuroscience-based studies supporting the idea that porn can be addictive.

Porn Facts

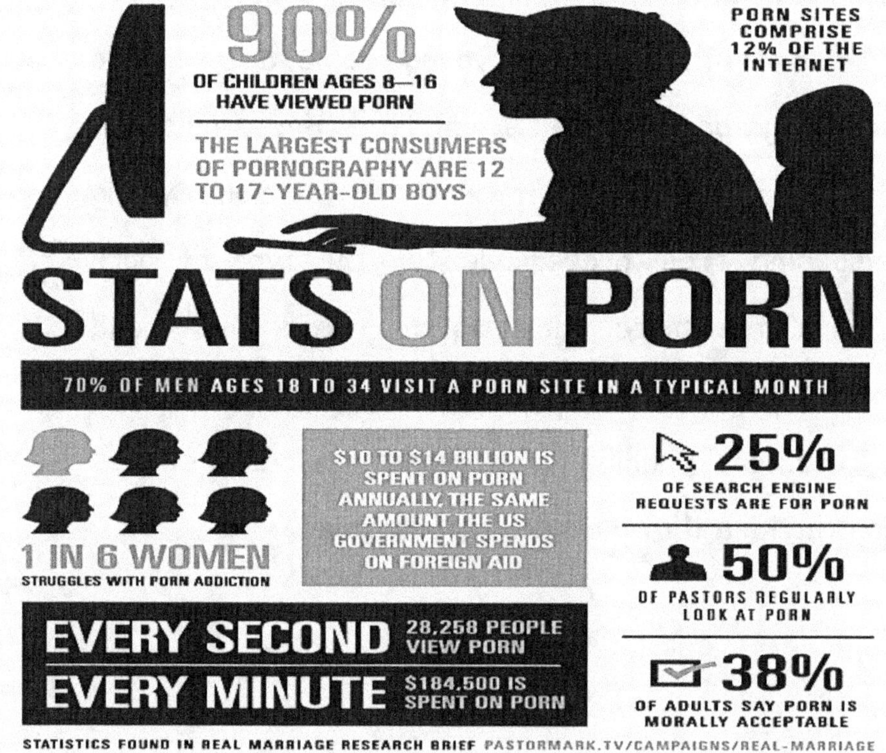

Strategies to Help Children with Pornography Addiction

The statistics can overwhelm any parent. Extremetech.com

estimates that about 30 percent of all data transferred

over the internet is pornography. It is found on literally hundreds of millions of web pages, including social media giants: Facebook, Twitter, YouTube. It is accessible through television, computers, tablets, and smartphones.

Here, I will be sharing with you eight strategies you can use to combat this. But first, take a look at these online porn statistics as recorded on www.therecoveryvillage.com:

- 30% of internet data is pornography
- 136 billion pornographic videos were viewed on smartphones in 2015
- Pornography is a $97 billion industry
- By comparison, the combined revenue of the top-10 sports leagues in North America, Europe, and Asia is $45.8 billion.

Here are eight strategies to help your child with overcoming pornography; adapted from the article *Arm Your Kids for the Battle* by Lisa Ann Thomson in BYU Magazine, Spring 2015.

1. Address Access and Family Rules

Simple steps and rules can protect children (and adults) from unintentional exposure and help them to think twice about the content they choose to view, such as:

- Use filters at the computer, router, and internet-service-provider levels
- Enable parental and content controls through cable providers and online media services
- Set up content restriction settings on mobile devices
- Keep computers and tablets in common areas
- Ask children and teens to turn in their phones and mobile devices at night
- Establish an open-book policy; parents can view texts and social media accounts at any time
- Teach children what to do if they stumble upon pornography:

i. Close their eyes and shut down the device

ii. Tell an adult

iii. Redirect their thoughts

iv. Assure them that they did nothing wrong and are not in trouble

2. Introduce Them to God

Experts agree that children understanding the true teaching of their religion is a good measure to lower or eliminate porn views. Studies have confirmed that religiosity in the home, coupled with a "warm parenting style," has a protective effect against pornography.

"The best preventative measure and the best reparative measure for pornography is the true teaching of the gospel in the home," says Timothy Rarick, parenting professor at Brigham Young University, Idaho, USA and member of the United Families International advisory board. "The best thing we can do is help our children establish their own connection to heaven."

3. Teach Children How to Filter Internally

As the world moves further and further away from the principles and guidelines given to us by God, we will stand out from the crowd. We will be different as we decide not to fill our minds with media choices that are base and demeaning and that will remove the Spirit from our homes and our lives.

Teach your teen to take responsibility for what he allows into his mind. His mind is like a garden, and what he feeds it with grows. This includes what he sees, reads, listens to or says when hanging out with friends.

Going forward, he needs to take value-based actions. He needs to ask himself:

- Why am I taking this action?
- What are the consequences?

- Will I be proud of myself if others, especially my parents, find out?

4. Teach Children Healthy Sexuality

The principle of "opposition in all things" applies to pornography. It is not enough to label pornography as bad; parents also need to teach their children what is good. One of the most powerful buffers and protections for our youth is to teach them sexuality in the home, starting early, young people   are suffering because they are growing up in a vacuum of toxic messages with too few positive messages within what is right according the gospel.

5. Shatter the Myth of Pornography

"Pornography use by adolescents and young adults often leads to a distorted view of sexuality and its role in fostering healthy personal relationships," points out the American College of Pediatricians. "These distortions include the overestimation of the prevalence of sexual activity in the community, the belief that sexual promiscuity is normal, and the belief that sexual abstinence is unhealthy."

In discussions about pornography, parents should point out that pornography is mythical on all levels. The behaviors portrayed in pornography are neither normal nor a reflection of what should be anticipated or expected in a healthy relationship. "Pornography is attractive only as long as the myth of pornography is embraced," Professor Carroll says.

6. Change the Conversation about the Problem

According to Professor Carroll, "Adolescents get involved with pornography out of curiosity, out of accessibility, and out of what, at its core, amounts to immaturity."

"Every one of us experiences the power of the sexual-response cycle triggered during puberty, long before we have the emotional or spiritual maturity to fully make sense of it. The problem is real and has terrible consequences, but making blanket statements about the problem often pushes it deeper into the souls of those struggling."

Pornography problems can range from "occasional or repeated intentional use, to intensive use, to compulsive (addictive) use. ... If behavior is incorrectly classified as an addiction, the user may think he or she has lost the capacity to overcome the problem. ... On the other hand, having a clearer understanding of the depth of the problem☐ – that it may not be as ingrained or extreme as feared☐ – can give hope and an increased capacity to ... repent."

When addressing issues on pornography, parents should take a triage approach

- How long has it been going on?
- How often do they view it?
- How are they accessing it?

Then parents can work with the teen to determine an appropriate level of action.

Understand the person and who they are:

- How deep is their problem?

- What is really going on?

- What is their reason for viewing pornography, and how can we address the deeper problems?

7. Teach Emotional Management

Addressing deeper problems is key to preventing pornography problems. Beyond natural curiosity, pornography is often used as a way to cope with emotions, particularly overwhelming emotion.

"At some point, a young man or woman has a difficult or distressing psychological, relational, or spiritual experience. Negative experiences can lead the adolescent brain to revert to 'feel-good experiences' such as viewing pornography and engaging in related behaviors such as masturbation. The emotions created in such behaviors then replace or mask distressing emotions. And therein lies the danger: the person moves away from a feel-good experience nto the initiation of a psychological dependency orientation. Now he or she is using the behavior as a way of managing life," says Professor Butler.

Parents should teach children that both pleasant and unpleasant emotions are normal, and it is okay to experience negative feelings such as sadness, anger, frustration, or hurt. Parents often feel the need to control their children's emotions, but allowing them to experience and cope with negative feelings builds a critical skill set.

If a pornography problem exists, parents should take care not to add to the child's emotional burden through shaming. School of family life professor James M. Harper noted that while guilt is a natural response to mistakes that can motivate change, shame is a destructive feeling that can lead to a sense of hopelessness. In other words, creating or exacerbating a feeling of shame in a child damages the child's ability both to develop positive emotional responses and to recognize the influence of the Spirit, which is ultimately the most powerful ally in the prevention of and recovery from pornography use.

A parent shared with me her struggles with her teen about porn and when we started working with this teenager we found out the mother's reaction made her feel worse. In her words, "My mother reacted strongly, yelling and screaming, and it made me feel worse about it, rather than hopeful of overcoming it."

8. Create a Plan for Your Child

It is important to recognize that when we fail to address pornography in the home, we may actually be teaching our children to not come to us when they encounter "forbidden" material online. Common reasons children give for withholding information from their parents include:

- Fear of getting in trouble
- Fear of disappointing their parents
- Lack of vocabulary to describe the problem
- Lack of understanding that they are in danger

On the other hand, when we do talk about pornography with our children we help them create a response in their brain that says 'Hey, this stuff is pornography, it's dangerous, you need to go tell a parent!'

Here is a story a parent who took the course we held on this subject in The Intentional Parent Academy shared with us:

I was just going through the introduction of porn literacy in the course "Walking Your Child Through Puberty" in the TIP Academy. Suddenly, it came like a flash where my own issues began. My cousin introduced me to porn videos when I was between 8-10 years old. I couldn't tell my parents. Even though I did not watch again, the images did not leave my mind and that led me into lesbianism.

By the time the caregiver who was living with us got to know and informed my parents, it was another terrible saga. My dad beat me up mercilessly. I was sleeping and he woke me up and beat me with his walking stick. I still have the marks on my thigh. But it still did not take the lesbianism away.

The funny thing is I was doing the despicable act with my younger sister who is 6 years younger than me. I struggled with it, I prayed, I tried to fight it many times and did everything and it still did not go away. It continued for 3-5 years.

One time I was caught again. We were in our own house then and my dad realized beating wasn't enough, so he took me to one of the rooms and locked me up there and told me that I wasn't going to come out of that room until I dealt with the shame. The first incident where he beat me up with his walking stick, he seized all my clothes and shoes and said he was going to take me to the river bank and throw me away, that I was a source of shame to him. He later gave me back everything after a while.

This time, in the room I was locked in I wasn't given food, only water for 3 days. At intervals he would come in and say some words over myself.

I was already having a good understanding of God at this age. I cried a lot in that room. I kept asking God "why me?" I wasn't enjoying it but I couldn't stop myself.

I continued like that for 3 days and he came at intervals and prayed with me. I decided that I wasn't going to do it again and told God it was only Him that could help me stop. And thanks to God, after that room it never happened again.

But when I got married it gave me a dysfunctional sex life. I didn't know how to explain the cause to my husband. It took time before it started getting better, and I won't even say I'm there yet. I'm still gradually building a normal sex life.

I'm sharing this with you because many parents don't understand the need to make this conversation open. Children need someone to talk to about it. Maybe if I was able to talk to my parents about what I watched, I wouldn't have gone that far. But the fear of how they would react that I'd already imagined in my mind made me get into a torment that tore me apart, the outcome of which I'm still trying to fix today.

I may not be able to share my story publicly, but you have a platform to share it. Please tell parents to let their children be able to talk to them. Thank you for all you do. When you said parenting is about me, I didn't fully understand it. When you said it was going to change me, I didn't get a hold of it; but with each step you guide us with on a daily basis, I'm visiting my past and I can see I'm getting better. I thank you for availing yourself to be used by God in this generation. I thank your husband for allowing you to thrive on this journey. I know God will reward you! I just wanted to say thank you. I'm really grateful.

** This was shared with me at the last batch of the course "Walking Your Child Through puberty"*

Sex Education is Porn Education

The average age today at which a child first views hardcore porn online is eight. Matter of fact, a Bitdefender survey conducted three years ago indicates that age could be as low as six. This isn't because 8 year olds and 6 year olds go ooking for porn; it's a function of what in today's digital world is inevitable and cannot be prevented, no matter how hard you try – they just stumble upon it somehow. So, just as you can't talk about sex too early to your child, you can't talk about porn too early either.

You could start thus: 'You know when we watch movies and TV together, we see things that aren't real, or things that are exaggerated and extreme? Well, that happens with sex too. People make movies and videos for entertainment that aren't real. These can be quite confusing and so it's a good idea not to watch them till you're older – but if you come across these or anyone shows you anything that confuses you, tell me/us and we can talk about it.'

Be explicit. Obviously, the degree of explicitness will vary with age, but parents need to be aware that however explicit they're being, kids are encountering far worse explicitness in the things they see online and being passed around by their friends. The most helpful thing you can do for your children is to be uncompromisingly straightforward. A friend of mine with teenagers said to me, "The world is so sexualized that if I don't teach my children about sex, the world will teach them what is against our family values."

Use outside prompts and the excellent resources that already exist. It's difficult for parents to embark on this dialogue out of nowhere; they need jumping off points. That can be anything: something that happens in a TV program or a movie, or something that comes up with one of your kids' friends. Use it as a springboard for discussion.

Must-Have Conversations on Porn

- Common porn related issues amongst students such as revenge porn, sexual pressure, pressure to watch porn and to send nudes
- Potential impacts of porn on students' sexual beliefs, attitudes and behaviours
- The new online porn landscape for students in terms of access, usage and content
- The need to build porn literacy skills in young people

Here is Why Porn Conversation is Key

- Social media as a sexualized environment

- There is high interest in sex during puberty

- Pornography and beliefs about sex

- Body image: sexual objectification can do a lot of harm to their sense of self-worth.

- Expectations around sex: pornography can influence a young person's expectations about sex; for example what young men expect their partners to do and vice versa. It can shape sexual practices.

How to Start the Porn Conversation

<u>Respect</u>:

Respect is an essential place to begin any conversation about porn. Explain that the disrespect men show towards women in porn isn't something that should be recreated or accepted. Talk about the fact that what they are seeing isn't real, that the people in the videos are paid actors.

Here are some simple tips for talking to teens about porn:

Get Prepared

Fact sheets about porn: a lot of young people watch porn to get ideas about sex and think it will make them better lovers. However, research shows us that using porn can have the opposite effect.

Prepare to be Un-Shockable

The chances are pretty high that the teen you are talking to has seen porn. Try not to act surprised about what they tell you, particularly if they talk about the type of porn they've seen. This isn't the time for shame and blame, so avoid words like bad or wrong and take a curious, open, non-judgmental approach.

Connection

Porn is a tough topic to bring up, so make sure you have a good rapport with the young person you're speaking with and that they feel safe with you.

I have advocated for a while now that parenting should be about connection. When I wrote my bestselling book *Connect to Correct*, it was inspired by the knowledge that before you can have these difficult conversations with a teen you will need a lot of connections. If you haven't started building a meaningful relationship with your child yet, you might want to get a copy of *Connect to Correct*, it will show you how to connect to the point that conversations like this won't be a problem.

Choose the Right Time, Place and Environment

Talking while doing an activity can work well as it can be less intense or confrontational. Some teens prefer to chat one to one, while others may like to talk in a group. Talking about porn with friends can be quite acceptable amongst some teens and doesn't have the same stigma it does for most adults.

Things to Consider

Some young people may have had negative experiences with porn and want to talk about it, but they're too embarrassed to raise it on their own. It's great to be aware of some of the common porn related issues that teens can face as you go into the conversation.

These can include...

- Feeling their porn use is out of control
- Seeking increasingly violent porn themes – and feeling uncomfortable with it, but unable to stop
- Having images of themselves sent around by friends or others and regretting it, but feeling too afraid to tell an adult
- Experiencing pressure to send nude photos
- Revenge porn (someone distributing nudes without consent)

- Feeling pressure to watch porn by friends

- Feeling upset, anxious or traumatized by images in porn, especially when there's a history of sexual abuse

(Check out the workbook for some conversation openers)

HOW DO I KNOW IF MY CHILD IS ALREADY VIEWING PORN?

I.   Your Child Spends Too Much Time Using Smart Devices

Did you know that only 13% of children use smartphones with parental restrictions? The rest are exposed to all kinds of content on the internet – unrestricted.[1]

There's a reason why tech innovators like Steve Jobs and Bill Gates banned cell phone access to their children until they were in their mid-teens. Smart devices can be addictive if not used with care. Studies as reported by commonsensemedia.org show that a staggering 82% of children and teenagers view pornography on smartphones and tablets.

Children nearing teenage have developing brains that find smartphones and adult content much more addictive as compared to a grown up. Once addicted, they can easily lose track of time and spend hours consuming illicit content.

Which is why if your children are spending more time than usual on the phone you should have a good look at their online activities and try to limit unnecessary access.

II.   Prefers Isolation and Spends Hours Behind Locked Doors

Excessive smartphone usage is usually followed by an increased preference for isolation. If that's happening to your child, don't ignore it, because it's a major warning sign that something's not right.

Children exposed to porn often have mixed feelings of excitement and shame. They feel a strong urge to view pornography when they're alone and look for ways to get away from their parents or guardians to a place where no one's watching. With time, this behavior intensifies and becomes a permanent personality trait even after children reach adulthood.

III.   Is Overprotective of His/Her Smart Devices

To keep them safe, young children should never be given access to smartphones without parental controls and clear media guidelines. Parents should be able to access their children's devices any time without any restrictions. However, that's often not the case with children who view pornography on their smartphones or tablets. In fact, such kids are usually overprotective of their phones and hesitate to allow access to anyone else.

If your child has suddenly added a security lock or password to his/her phone and keeps it close to themselves all the time (even when going to the toilet) you should intervene.

IV.   Stays Quiet, Depressed and Uninterested in the Outside World

The relationship between depression, anxiety and pornography is pretty well documented. This mainly has to do with how viewing porn frequently alters the human brain.

These effects are exaggerated in children because their brains are still developing and more vulnerable to the extreme emotions that a person experiences while viewing porn. As a result, the affected child experiences depression and a general lack of motivation about everything in life.

V.   Has Irregular Sleep Cycles and Struggles to Get Up in the Morning

If your child has access to their smartphone and the internet even in the bedroom, then you need to keep a close eye on their sleep patterns and energy levels in the morning.

According to research, most people log in to porn sites after midnight on weekends and after 10.00 PM on weekdays. Bedtime porn consumption can go on for hours because there's nothing else left to do in the day and no one is watching. When that happens, a child may experience lack of sleep, headache, and may struggle to get out of bed in the morning. If you see this happening regularly, or notice your child sleeping at odd times of the day, you must look into the matter with more concern.

VI.   Panics and Changes Online Activities If You
Suddenly Show Up

How does your child react if you suddenly enter his/her
bedroom, walk up to them or ask to use their smartphone?
Does he/she panic, stop what they're doing and appear
nervous? If yes, it might be a good idea to actually see
what's running on that device.

It's a natural reaction since most children who watch porn
realize that their parents won't be happy to know about it.

VII. Has   Started   Struggling   at   Studies   and
Extracurricular Activities

Falling grades, deteriorating academic performance, and a
general preference for smartphones or tablets over
extracurricular activities are some of the major signs of
porn consumption in children.

Researchers at the National Center for Biotechnology
Information, USA (NCBI) found that the working memory of

children and teenagers who regularly viewed porn deteriorated over time. Such children also suffered from lack of motivation and found it hard to compete with their peers. As a result, they were much more likely to stay away from outdoor games and competitive activities that are crucial for personality development.

VIII. Can't Concentrate for Long and has Sudden Mood Swings

The loss of working memory, which I just mentioned above, also has a direct impact on a child's ability to concentrate on a task or assignment. This is why children who are exposed to porn early in their lives often find it hard to perform mind-intensive tasks.

This can also lead to sudden mood swings, unnecessary aggression and other forms of erratic behavior in children. Look out for these changes in your child and see if they're connected in any way with his/her smartphone usage habits.

IX. Has Increased Interest in Sexual Topics, Discussions, and Content

Sex is a fascinating topic for teenagers (and even young children) and it's common for them to talk about it with friends. But if your child suddenly starts taking a lot more interest in sex-related TV programs or frequently mentions sexual terminologies in conversations, it's a clear red flag that shouldn't go unnoticed.

Check out the workbook for some conversation openers:

How Do I Know If My Child is Already Viewing Porn?

Check out the workbook on porn conversations for details

PROTECT YOUR CHILDREN FROM UNWANTED SEXUAL CONTENT

Internet porn is a reality that you cannot change or runaway from. You also can't disconnect your children from the world and completely deprive them of the knowledge and the learning resources available on the internet. But you can keep a close eye on their activities, guide them about internet usage, and protect them from any content that can have detrimental effects on their minds and personalities by using adult filters and strict parental controls.

Trust your children, but don't leave them unguarded on the internet because, as I mentioned at the start, most children are exposed to sexual content for the first time by accident. So, make sure your child browses the internet without any surprises.

Chapter 5

TECH CONVERSATIONS?

Parents worry about TV and game additions, but what we are faced with today is more! Phones, tablets, apps, social media, texting all captivate kids (and adults), starting at a very young age.

We are now faced with questions like:

- When is the right time to give my kids their first gadget?
- Will they be able to manage one properly?
- Will it soon be a tool of distraction?
- How am I sure my teen will be safe online?

These and more are the questions parents ask in a bid to assure the safety of their child/teen online. But then, who is satisfactorily answering these all-important questions?

Why You Must Have the Tech Conversation

- The tech conversation gives you the leverage to reinforce your family values in your child

- It sets the tone of your teen's relationship with technology and their use of devices

- It helps you to educate your tweens and teens on the world of the web, their online safety, how they can make technology work for them and not otherwise.

The internet is the new teacher who has no filter. This means that with just a tab children have access to a world of limitless information – good and bad. Today, children don't bother asking their parents or even teachers questions. Like adults, if they have access to the internet, they just ask 'Google', and they get served a 'buffet' of options.

This brings to the fore the question of values: where will your children learn the most important life lessons – from you or the internet?

The tech conversation in this regard will help parents prepare their children for the diverse knowledge available online and how they can filter what they should learn or not, believe or not.

Teen-related Tech Realities

#1:   Today's teens spend more time online than ever before

#2:   Teens know a lot more about technology than most adults

#3:   Teens have the power to build a positive online reputation and become good digital citizens

When to Have Tech Conversations

I am of the opinion that tech conversations should start from day one, even before your child can own a personal device. Before your teen gets her first gadget or starts using any app at all, including social media, it is vital to have 'the tech conversation' with them.

Tech conversations refer to various engagements, conversations and actions taken to educate your children about gadgets, the world of web, do's and don'ts, how to have a healthy relationship with and make the most of technology. The tech conversation isn't just a conversation, that is what you say to your child; it involves how you model technology/gadget use, build boundaries, spend time on apps/platforms, and more. In essence, it starts from Day 0, when your child can watch and learn from you.

The Tech conversation isn't a one-time conversation. It will happen over time and at different ages of your child, given different scenarios. Parents must learn to maximize what I call 'teachable moments' to engage their kids accordingly.

Watch things together. Screen time can be an opportunity for family bonding. At this time, important conversations, building healthy boundaries and communicating clear values can take place.

Ask them questions during your watch or afterwards. Let them share their thoughts on certain scenes, characters, or lessons learnt.

Listen to their opinions and share your informed or value-based perspective as well. If you're worried that your kids are getting wrong messages from the media, the best way to counteract them is to have screen time alongside your kids.

Don't make screens a reward in your home. Technology is enormously appealing to teens as it is. When we make screen time the go-to thing kids get for good behaviour – or get taken away for bad behaviour – we are making it even more desirable, thereby increasing the chances that a child will overvalue it.

Encourage other activities. There are many ways to have fun. Running around outside, playing a sport, reading books, doing crafts, etc. Variety is vital for a balanced life. Encourage your children to develop a wide range of interests. Model doing so yourself. Let your children see you reading a book, making things and having a hobby (or some). Finally, present these activities as equally rewarding as screen time – not alternatives to it.

TECH CONVERSATIONS START WITH YOU

It is really great that you are thinking and talking about this important subject of modeling screen time to your children. It is a right step in the right direction. However, a major problem with the goal of "trying to model better" lies in the ambiguity of the goal – and ambiguous goals never go well.

Consider asking yourself these questions sincerely:

- How do I model screen time in my home?
- What messages do my actions with my devices signal to my child?
- Have my children seen me try to change a habit, screen time, or others?
- Do I use the SMART approach to behavior change?
- Is there anything around my screen time habits that I think I should consider changing?

Rather than having a vague goal like "I should model screen time better," pick a *specific* goal and model how you are going to try to reach that goal. Helping your teen learn skills around behavior change through one's own efforts is such a valuable gift to them.

A goal can be even something like changing the type of shows one decides to watch. Yes, as simple as that.

Examples of parents setting specific goals:

i. After checking my email, my goal is to turn off the WiFi on my computer for one hour each weekday morning so I can get my writing done and not get tempted to check my email repeatedly or social media feeds and notifications.

ii. I am going to try to resist checking my phone when we are setting up for dinner and at the table, so I get to talk with my family in a more connected way.

iii. My goal is to only check my social media handles for 1hour in a day.

iv. My goal is to take a full weekend off screens this month and see how I feel afterward.

v.   I plan to no longer have my phone in my room at night, just like I have decided I don't want my teens to have theirs.

vi.   I plan to delete my favorite sports app off my phone because I check it too often. I want to see if I can keep it off permanently and only look up sports on my computer.

A Model for Effective Behavior Change

If you have a desired change that you would consider announcing and trying, there is a model for behavior change I love in Joshua Klapow's book *Living Smart*.

S   -   Set a reasonable, small, and actionable goal.

M   -   Monitor your progress by doing something   like noting on a calendar each time you succeed.

A   - Arrange for success, like put the book you   want to read by your bedside so that you're ready to go the evening your screen-free night/weekend arrives.

R   -   Recruit people to help hold you accountable.

Tell your children, husband, wife, or some friends about your goal and ask them to ask you about it every now and then. Wanting the ego-lift of being able to report success can give you some extra motivation. Honestly though, knowing that your children were witnesses to any attempts can be the strongest motivation. And if you slip, ask them for their suggestions of what you could do better. Trust me, they would love giving you advice.

T   -   Treat.

Choose a personal reward you value, like having a special dessert. All the data shows that sustained behavior change comes when we get rewards for our change. For example, if one does not like the gym where they do the elliptical, over time they will stop going. But if they allow themselves to watch their favorite show only when they are on the elliptical, it can be enough of a reward that they stick with it. Or, they get the reward that they actually start to enjoy the movement of an elliptical.

What About Tech Must You Discuss?

I.   What is your child sharing online?

Posting something online can be compared to getting a tattoo; once you press 'send' it's out there for the world to see. Sometimes, like a tattoo, the online content we post can be covered up or removed. However, that too, can be time consuming, costly and/or painful. This is why we need to constantly remind our children, especially our teenagers, to think before they post. It's also why we need to start having conversations early about privacy and reputation.

II.   Privacy

Privacy! Does your child understand this? A recent PEW study revealed that 81% of parents of teens give too much information to online advertisers. We have to set an example for our children. Do your children know never to give out their full name, address, phone number or other private information online? I know it sounds simple, but take a look at digital kidnapping these days where identity can be falsified and stolen and, worse, it can pose a risk of real kidnapping for the child or their parent.

Familiarize yourself with the types of information being collected on the sites your child uses and have a conversation with them about what is and isn't okay to share. Let's remind our children they are in control of their information and have the power to decide what the internet knows about them.

III.   Reputation

How to differentiate between public and private isn't the only conversation we need to have when teaching our children to think before they press 'send'. We also need to talk about online reputation. Do your children understand that they are painting a picture about themselves with every interaction they have online – pictures that can easily be found by business partners, nations and even recruiters or future employers? Telling them this isn't meant to scare them. Rather, it's meant to serve as a reminder to pay attention to what they are doing. It can also serve as a reminder for how much opportunity they have to turn their reputation into a masterpiece! They get to decide what the world sees online and they have the chance to make it something wonderful.

I know a lot parents feel stressed by the technology that's out there and these types of conversations. From social media and apps to music players and video games, the cyberspace is massive and grows larger every day. But it's absolutely critical that parents try to stay ahead of their kids, technically speaking. I know sometimes that's not realistic, so if not ahead of our kids, let's at least try to catch up. If your child or teen is on a website or social networking site you are not familiar with, learn about it! Think of it as if your child is going to visit a new neighbor. Wouldn't you want to meet them and know who they are hanging out with beforehand?

While technology absolutely has its risks, we can empower our children to understand and overcome the downsides. Parents and children can work together to build important skills. That way, though the internet never sleeps, we can give them the tools to succeed and we can all sleep more peacefully.

Chapter 6
FACTS ABOUT LGBT

LGBTQ is an acronym for Lesbian, Gay, Bisexual, Transgender and Queer or Questioning. These terms are used to describe a person's sexual orientation or gender identity.

Whereas, LGBPTTQQIIAA+ (Alphabet Soup) is any combination of letters attempting to represent all the identities in the queer community. This near-exhaustive one (but not exhaustive still) represents Lesbian, Gay, Bisexual, Pansexual, Transgender, Transsexual, Queer, Questioning, Intersexual, Intergender, Asexual, Ally.

With respect to LGBTQ sexual relations, the age of consent in the United Kingdom was lowered to sixteen. It is fourteen in Canada, fifteen in Sweden, fifteen in France, fourteen in Germany, Iceland, Italy, San Marino, and Slovenia; twelve in Spain, Holland, Malta, and Portugal. Isn't it utterly outrageous that twelve-year-olds in these latter countries, most of whom will not have reached puberty, can give their consent to older males or females who want to exploit them sexually? Furthermore, their parents can't legally prevent the exploitation. The question that jumps out at us is, "Why have gay and lesbian organizations worked feverishly to lower the age of accountability?" James Dobson asks in his book *Raising Boys*.

I shared statistics somewhere and a renowned lawyer noted that it's 11 years in Nigeria, since a girl can marry at same age. I know many parents are still ignorant of the fact that the LGBTQ is not visible in this part of the world and there are lots of support system making this even gain more grounds. One factor I have seen that has given this wings to fly is that teenagers never get the required support on the issue of their sexuality in their teen years.

Sexual Orientation During Puberty

Homosexuality is *not* normal and should not be thought of or taught as "normal." Throughout adolescence, most youth will question their sexual orientation in one way or another. This can be a confusing time, but that's why they have parents to guide them, to sufficiently connect with them so as to help them through that phase of life and into responsible adulthood.

But first, what do you as a parent need to know about LGBT?

No 'gay gene'.

The largest study till date on the genetic basis of sexuality has revealed five spots on the human genome that are linked to same-sex sexual behaviour, but none of the markers are reliable enough to predict someone's sexuality.

In 1993, geneticist Dean Hamer of the U.S. National Cancer Institute and his colleagues published a paper suggesting that an area on the X chromosome called Xq28 could contain a "gay gene." But other studies, found no such link.

Throughout Europe, being gay or lesbian is legal. However, there is an "East/West" divide on further LGBTQ rights.

- In May of 2017, Taiwan became the first Asian country to legalize same-sex marriage.
- In Japan, the LGBTQ market is worth an estimated US$600 billion.
- Guyana is the only country in South and Latin America where homosexuality is illegal and punishable by prison.
- In 2013, Uruguay passed the same-gender marriage laws by a large majority.
- Same-sex marriage is legal in Canada.
- South Africa is the only country in Africa where same-gender marriage is legal.
- Approximately 1 million children in the U.S. are being raised by same-sex couples.

Do you know Facebook has 58 gender options for users to choose from?

Overwhelming right? Knowledge is a prerequisite for parenting the 21st Century child.

How to Talk to Your Child about LGBTQ

The reality is if you don't, someone else probably will – or already is. And you may not like what they have to say.

Homosexuality has become increasingly visible in our culture, moving from acceptance and normalization to celebration and promotion. This is happening in every area of life, from education to entertainment, from the media to the marketplace, and from cities and counties to courts and churches.

Think about the tremendous changes we've seen in this regard:

- 1997 was the year comedienne Ellen DeGeneres "came out" and was featured on the cover of Time magazine.
- 2004 was the year "same-sex marriage" was ordered by the Supreme Court of Massachusetts, the first state to redefine marriage.

- "Glee" premiered on television in 2009, with a storyline focusing on a male character identifying as gay.
- 2012 was when President Barack Obama finally "evolved" on the issue of marriage, fully supporting its redefinition to include two men or two women.

And today?

Christians who believe God's design for marriage and sexuality are routinely labeled and assumed to be "haters," "homophobes" and "bigots." Some want to keep our view out of the public square.

Christian parents face many questions, such as:

- How do I talk to my children about homosexuality?
- How do I protect their innocence but also prepare them for the world around them?
- How do I build into them a biblical worldview of gender and sexuality?"

Countering Confusion

For parents discussing homosexuality for older children, we have shared conversation starters you can use to engage them. Refer to chapter 6 of the Workbook.

Chapter 7
DRUG CONVERSATIONS

Sometime ago I shared a research statistic by the National Drug Law Enforcement Agency (NDLEA) in our Facebook community, which says that by 2025 one in every 5 homes in Nigeria will have a drug user. That post was met with a lot of frantic prayers of 'It's not my portion; God forbid!' as response.

As much as I too would love to say 'God forbid!' and go to sleep, the sad reality is that 'God forbid!' only is not a parenting strategy; we need education and strategy on exactly what to do and how. But unfortunately, many parents stop at just mumbling those empty words and continue parenting as though it's business as usual.

Parents who are educated about the effects of drug use and learn the facts can give their children correct information and clear up any misconceptions. You're a role model for your child, and your views on alcohol, tobacco and drugs can strongly influence how they think about them. So, make talking about drugs a part of your general health and safety conversations with your children. Just as you protect your kids against illnesses like measles, you can help "immunize" them against drug use by giving them the facts before they're in a risky situation.

When kids don't feel comfortable talking to their parents, they'll seek answers elsewhere, even if their sources are unreliable. And kids who aren't properly informed are at greater risk of engaging in unsafe behaviors and experimenting with drugs.

Not long ago, I counselled a 23-year-old graduate from a Christian university who told me that 80% of students in her school do drugs and it's not really a big deal. Over the past year alone, nearly 15% of the adult population in Nigeria (around 14.3 million people) reported a "considerable level" of use of psychoactive drug substances – it's a rate much higher than the 2016 global average of 5.6% among adults. The survey was led by Nigeria's National Bureau of

Statistics (NBS) and the Center for Research and Information on Substance Abuse with technical support from the United Nations Office on Drugs and Crime (UNODC) and funding from the European Union.

According to UNODC, in Nigeria, one in seven persons aged 15-64 years had used a drug (other than tobacco and alcohol) in the past year. The past year prevalence of any drug use is estimated at 14.4 per cent (range: 14.0 per cent - 14.8 per cent), corresponding to 14.3 million people aged 15-64 years who had used a psychoactive substance in the past year for non-medical purposes.

In a world drug report by the UNODC in 2019, people worldwide who had used opioids – a class of drugs naturally found in the opium poppy plant – had surged by 56 per cent, and this was attributed to improved knowledge of the extent of drug use from new surveys conducted in two highly populated countries, namely India and Nigeria.

Millennials – people born in the 1980s, 1990s or early 2000s – the architects of the Nigerian future, are full of adventure and willing to try new things, however, this same fearless adventurism makes them the perfect target for hard drug experimentation and eventual dependency. Aggravating the situation are the manners and genres of music that influence the youth and have a negative effect on their behaviour, schoolwork, social interactions and mood. Music lyrics that glorify drugs, sex and violence have become the order of the day.

The perceptions and effects of music-video messages are important as exposure to violence, sexual messages and stereotypes, and use of substances of abuse in music videos might produce significant changes in behaviours and attitudes of young viewers. Also, the low investment in treatment and care for people with drug use disorders complicates matters for those carried away by this perception.

Furthermore, there is a strong correlation between drug addiction, rape and crime. Combating drug addiction and trafficking in Nigeria is a good first step to ending the menace of rapes and crimes in the country.

It has been observed that the high rate of drug addiction in Nigeria has continued unabated as at least 7,800 people are introduced to drug abuse daily. This revelation was made by a health practitioner and President, Health Promoters and Awareness Initiative, Malam Saraki Abubakar Musa. According to him, the recent research conducted on the prevalence of hard drugs abuse revealed that 7,800 new cases are being recorded daily across the country, adding that 54 per cent of drug addicts are adolescent children from the age of 18 and below. Musa explained that the drugs mostly abused include tobacco, alcohol, synthetic drugs, ecstasy, cocaine, crystal meth and methamphetamine, inhalants, heroin and others, pointing out that "peer pressure and depression are causes of drug addiction among youths." He added, "Youths associate with different types of people otherwise known as friends. Through the pressure from these friends, a child may end up having a taste of these drugs, and once this is done they continue to take it and become addicted."

Collectively, smoking, alcohol and illicit drug use kill 11.8 million people each year. This is more than the number of deaths from all cancers! Let me reiterate: drug use is directly and indirectly responsible for 11.8 million deaths each year. In other words, smoking, alcohol and drug use are an important risk factor for early, premature death.

GETTING THE DRUG CONVERSATION STARTED

Start Now

It is never too early to talk to your children about alcohol and other drugs. Children as young as 9 years old already start viewing alcohol in a more positive way, and approximately 3,300 kids as young as 12 try marijuana each day. Additionally, about 5 in 10 kids as young as 12 obtain prescription pain relievers for nonmedical purposes (UNODC, 2018). The earlier you start talking, the better.

Plan Your Conversation

Plan a quiet time with your child when neither of you will have other distractions. You may go for a walk, plan an outing or chat in the car on the way home from school. It might also be useful to use cues from relevant topics on the

TV or in the media. You can start the conversation with some basic information.

Explain that a drug can be natural – such as cannabis or tobacco, or manufactured – such as ecstasy and ice. Let your child know that every drug changes our physical and psychological state in some way.

Explain that drugs fall into three groups:

- Everyday substances such as coffee or prescription medication
- Legal recreational drugs such as cigarettes and alcohol
- Illegal drugs such as speed, cocaine, ice and ecstasy

Explain that people use drugs (or medications) for different reasons:

- To treat illness
- To feel relief from pain
- To feel 'up' and energetic
- To feel relaxed and calm
- To fall asleep

From this information, your child will probably have questions. Let the conversation flow from those questions. In other words, let the conversation go in whatever direction your child wants to take it. You can always come back to your prepared information on another day. Remember it is also important to gauge your child's views about drugs and alcohol, and to talk about what they would do in different situations.

Lay Good Groundwork

No parent, child, or family is immune to the effects of drugs. Any kid can end up in trouble, even those who have made an effort to avoid it and even when they have been given the proper guidance from their parents.

However, certain groups of kids may be more likely to use drugs than others. Kids who have friends who use drugs are likely to try drugs themselves. Those feeling socially isolated for whatever reason may turn to drugs. So, it's important to know your child's friends – and their parents. Be involved in your children's lives. If your child's school runs an anti-drug program, get involved. You might learn something! Pay attention to how your kids are feeling and let them know that you're available and willing to listen in a nonjudgmental way. Recognize when your kids are going through difficult times so that you can provide the support they need or seek additional care if it's needed.

Role-play

Role-playing can help your child develop strategies to turn down drugs if they are offered. Act out possible scenarios they may encounter. Helping them construct phrases and responses to say no prepares them to know how to respond before they are even in that situation.

A warm, open family environment where children can talk about their feelings, where their achievements are praised, and where their self-esteem is boosted encourages kids to come forward with their questions and concerns. When censored in their own homes, kids go elsewhere to find support and answers to their most important questions.

Make talking and having conversations with your kids a regular part of your day. Finding time to do things you enjoy together as a family helps everyone stay connected and maintain open communication.

Chapter 8

SUPPORTING YOUR CHILD DURING PUBERTY

◻

WHEN TO START TALKING

Most parents don't think of puberty until they start to see changes in their own child or in their child's friends. Or they think of it as 'The Talk,' that is *one* big talk where you tell your kids everything they need to know in one long drawn-out conversation. We now know that 'the talk' doesn't work and that kids learn better from having many open and honest ongoing conversations. Which means that parents need to be having many conversations about puberty and not just *the one*!

So, what does this look like in the everyday home?

It might mean your 7-year-old walks into the bathroom whilst you're changing your tampon and asks, 'Why are you bleeding?' And you tell them that it's called a period, that it's normal and is something that happens to all girls when they grow up.

Or your 11-year-old asks if she can wear a bra because all her friends are starting to wear them. And you talk about the fact that puberty starts at a different time for everyone and that when she starts to grow breasts she too can and will wear a bra.

By answering your child's questions and talking about puberty openly and honestly, you are letting your child know that puberty will one day happen to them. You're also normalizing it and making puberty sound like an everyday thing, instead of something to be afraid of.

WHAT TO DO

One of the best strategies to employ during your child's puberty is reassurance. Explain that puberty is an exciting time that means adulthood is approaching.

<u>Compassion</u>

Try to show compassion for the changes they're experiencing and reassure them the changes are normal – and many will pass. Of course, if you're concerned about your child's development in any area, talk to a professional.

Role-Model Body Acceptance

Puberty is also a time when role-modelling body acceptance is really valuable. Your child will compare their body to those of their friends and may feel worried about their own development. The best thing you can do is show understanding and explain that bodies come in all shapes and sizes. Modelling a healthy lifestyle will also help your child.

Teens often make snap decisions, leading to risky behaviours. Expand their range of options and teach them to consider multiple choices and to weigh the potential risks and benefits of each decision. During this time, it's important to help your teen understand that emotions, good or bad, may affect their ability to make rational decisions.

Give Objective Information

Teens are often influenced by social pressures from other teens, which can lead them to participate in risky behaviours. Instead of imposing your opinions on your teen, provide them with objective information about these behaviours.

Although during the teen years there is often less time being spent with family, family closeness is still an extremely important component of adolescent development and has been associated with a lower incidence of smoking, alcohol and drug usage, and suicide attempts.

<u>Have Conversations; Don't Pressure</u>

Simply asking questions and listening without judgment can be majorly influential. Ask non-threatening questions that help them define their identities, such as:

- Who do you admire and why?
- What are your hopes for the future?
- What are your strengths?

To create a nonjudgmental environment, listen more than you speak. Ask open-ended questions to encourage them to think through their answers as opposed to just saying yes or no. Match their mood to help your teen feel like you understand where they are coming from.

<u>Uphold Family Values</u>

Concerns about popularity and acceptance are most intense during the early teen years and may lead teens to participate in risky behaviours. Parents can help teens resist these pressures and find alternative groups. Explain your family's set of values, like respecting yourself and others, the importance of trust, etc. If your family does not have some values central in the lives of your children, you should create some immediately and start using them to teach.

Sometime in 2020 I created a template that can help families build their family values without hassles. You can get a copy on my website: www.wendyologe.com

Additional Tips

- Praise your teenager for their efforts, achievements and positive behaviour.

- Put yourself in your child's shoes and try to see their behaviour for what it often is: your child struggling to become an individual personality.

- Try to stay calm during angry outbursts from your child. Wait for your child to cool down before talking about the problem. You can get a copy of my book *The Discipline That Works* to help you learn more on discipline.

- Stay interested and involved, and be available if your child wants to talk.

- Chat with your spouse or other parents of teenagers. Sharing concerns and experiences can ease the load.

- Try to support your child in their self-expression, even if some of it seems odd to you, such as an extreme haircut or offbeat clothing choices.

- Try to tolerate long periods of time spent on personal care, such as hours in the bathroom, but chat with your child about reasonable family time limits.

- Talk with your child about any permanent changes they want to make to their body, such as tattoos and piercings, and discuss temporary alternatives, such as henna (removable) tattoos.

- If your child has acne, talk with them on how they feel about it. If it is bothering them, ask if they would like to see a doctor. Your doctor may refer your teenager to a skin specialist or dermatologist.

HOW YOU CAN SUPPORT YOUR DAUGHTER

- Helping your daughter with firsts, such as being ready for her first period, are really important. Discreetly pack some sanitary items in her schoolbag and explain to her how to use them; for example, not sleeping with a tampon in place.

- Be ready for period pain: a hot water bottle and pain relief from your doctor or pharmacist may help. Talk to your doctor if your daughter hasn't had her period by 16 or 17 years of age, or if her periods stop after they've started.

- Remember, explain to your daughter that all these changes are natural and happen to every girl in her own time.

HOW YOU CAN SUPPORT YOUR SON

- Helping your son through puberty is mostly about reassurance. Reassure your son that testes develop unevenly and it's common for one to be lower than the other. If your son's testes are very small or not both in the scrotum, see your GP (General Practitioner).

- You may also need to reassure your son that penis size does not affect sexual functioning, and that erect penises are usually very similar in size. Every boy develops in his own time. Ejaculating during sleep (sometimes called a wet dream) and spontaneous erections are both normal.

- If your son experiences breast growth or tenderness, he may be concerned. Again, reassurance is the key. Any tenderness is likely to settle once his chest widens. If your son feels small or too thin for his age, reassure him he will grow in time.

- Remember, you know your child best. If anything about their development concerns you, see your Doctor.

Chapter 9

WHAT YOUR CHILD MIGHT STRUGGLE WITH

We all agree that puberty is a time of real struggle for your child. So it is worthy of note that as their body is going through a lot of changes they won't only battle with physical changes, they will also battle with their emotions, their mental health and their spirituality.

Here are some of the things you should look at for.

BODY IMAGE

The best time to talk about puberty with your child is before it begins. Take an open and relaxed approach to chatting with your child. Use the correct terms for body parts so your child learns the right words and is comfortable using them when talking about their body. They need to know their body parts are normal and natural, with words to match.

You may like to open a conversation by asking whether your child has learned about puberty at school and what they've been taught. Convey facts in the conversation, such as 'Every kid goes through these changes, but not always at the same time. Have you noticed that?' And talk about your values too.

INDEPENDENCE

It's normal for your child to want more independence – but still need your support – during puberty or teen years. They may take risks as they explore their boundaries and potentials.

As a parent, you may be worried about your child's safety and find yourself arguing with them about their push for independence. Try to stay calm and work through the issues with your child instead. Communicate openly and make sure your child knows you're there for them. Stay available, because being accessible is the best way to find out what your child is doing and to help keep them safe.

Talk to your child about making good decisions and your family's values. Ask your child to be comfortable and responsible to tell you where they are and what they're doing per time.

SOCIAL MEDIA

The internet, mobile phones and social media can influence how your child communicates with friends and learns about the world. Teach your child before the world will teach them!

MASTURBATION

Many boys will start wanting to experiment on masturbating more when they reach puberty. That is because they will have more erections at this time. Erections occur when blood rushes to the penis and causes it to harden. Erections are normal. Erections can happen at any time. They can occur with or without arousal. Masturbation can lead to a feeling of pleasure and relaxation.

An erection can happen during sleep. Sometimes, a boy will wake up with wet sheets due to semen being released (ejaculated) from the penis while asleep. Semen is a fluid that contains sperm. Ejaculating while asleep is common and normal.

Puberty involves heightened release of hormones in the body. There will be new feelings towards peers and sexual curiosity. Your son may have sexual thoughts or feelings. Many of his peers will talk about sex. They may have sex.

Start conversations early on sex education. Teach your child to internalize. Teach them that this feeling is normal and create distractive ways to expel this energy. Many of these come through the thought process and the mind.

PORN

Here's the problem: exposure to a sexual culture causes boys and girls to become consumers of people. It puts them on a path towards distorted love and disrespect of others. Pornography, sexual fantasies and sexual talk becomes the norm.

Pornography is powerful and creates a desire for more. It's far more pervasive than you would suspect. The rise of social media, sexting and technology in general has created soft landing for both boys and girls to get hooked on pornographic content and experiences.

Silence is not an option

Unfortunately, this is a topic we, parents, need to address with our kids. But rather than just saying no to porn and sexual fantasy, let's help our kids understand why it's so dangerous.

CONCLUSION

Walking Your Child Through Puberty is a book that has taken me years to publish and I believe reading it was worth your time.

Remember, start that conversation today. Puberty is progressive!

Congratulations.

Connect with The Parent Coach, ***Wendy Ologe:***

The Intentional Parent Academy

Facebook   Wendy Onyenezi-Ologe

Facebook page   Wendy Ologe-Theintentionalparent

Instagram   wendyologe or theintentionalparents

Twitter   ologewendy

Website   www.wendyologe.com
                      www.theintentionalparentacademy.com

Email   theintentionalparents@gmail.com

Mobile/WhatsApp   +2348034377085

www.ingramcontent.com/pod-product-compliance
Lightning Source LLC
Chambersburg PA
CBHW061349250726

48657CB00004B/1406